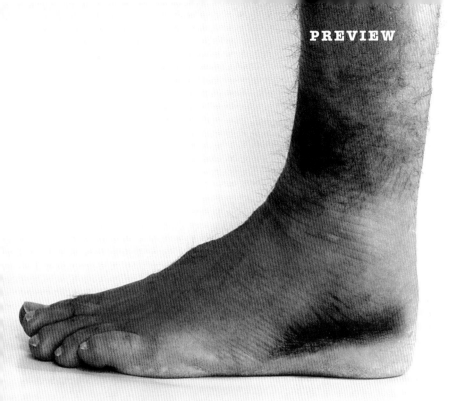

It started as a simple bruise on Bo Salisbury's ankle. But before long, his leg was killing him. Literally.

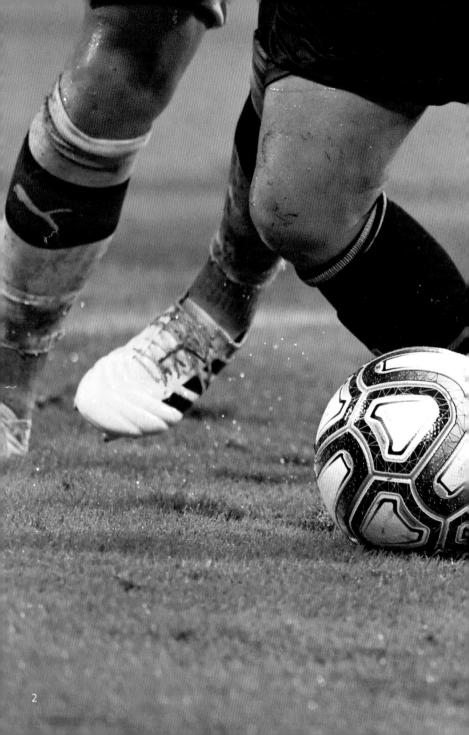

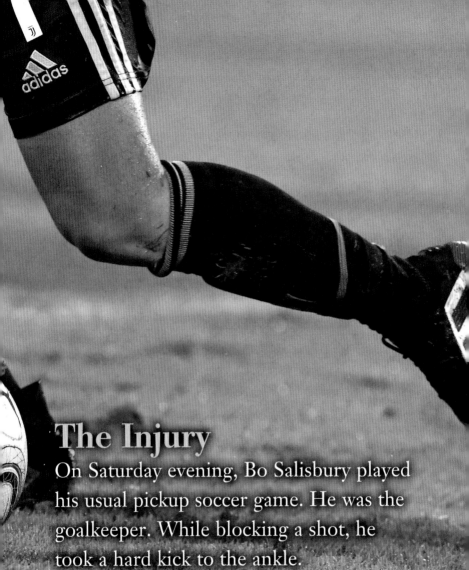

The Injury

On Saturday evening, Bo Salisbury played his usual pickup soccer game. He was the goalkeeper. While blocking a shot, he took a hard kick to the ankle.

It hurt, but Salisbury didn't worry about it.

The Symptoms

On Sunday, Salisbury's ankle was swollen and throbbing with pain. A doctor gave him painkillers. They didn't help.

By Monday, Salisbury had developed a fever. He was rushed to the hospital, where he began to slip in and out of consciousness.

He thought he was going to die. He said good-bye to his family.

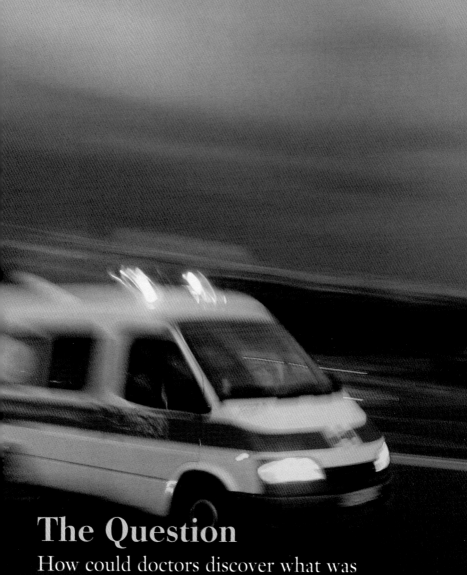

The Question

How could doctors discover what was wrong with Salisbury? And what would it take for him to win the fight for his life?

Cover design: Maria Bergós, Book&Look **Interior design:** Red Herring Design/NYC

Photo Credits ©: 1 top: Gary Lawton/Alamy Images; 8: Chris Bjornberg/Science Source; 13: Phanie/Science Source; 14: RapidEye/Getty Images; 18: Blend Images/Alamy Images; 20: Courtesy of Dr. Susan Murin; 22: Wavebreakmedia Ltd/Dreamstime; 23 top: Custom Medical Stock Photo/Alamy Images; 23 right top: Tim Vernon, LTH NHS Trust/Science Source; 24: Dr. Kenneth Greer/Getty Images; 27: Barry Slaven/Medical Images; 28 center: Gianni Dagli Orti/Shutterstock; 28 bottom: Hulton Archive/Getty Images; 29 top left: Mary Evans Picture Library/age fotostock; 29 center: Alfred Pasieka/Science Source; 29 bottom: Everett Collection/Shutterstock; 33: Vance Salisbury/Dr. Susan Murin/www.flesheatingbacteria.net; 34: PeopleImages/Getty Images; 36: Mike Devlin/Science Source; 38: Courtesy of Dr. Rekha Murthy, M.D.; 39: AJPhoto/Science Source; 41 top left: Comstock Images/Alamy Images; 41 top right: Corbis Premium Collection/Alamy Images; 41 bottom left: Reza Estakhrian/Getty Images; 42 cellulitis: Dr P. Marazzi/Science Source; 42 boils: SPL/Science Source; 42 scalded skin: Dr M.A. Ansary/Science Source.

All other photos © Shutterstock.

With thanks to Thomasine E. Lewis Tilden

Library of Congress Cataloging-in-Publication Data
Names: Phillips, Shea, author.
Title: Flesh wound : a minor injury takes a deadly turn / Shea Phillips.
Description: [New edition] | New York : Children's Press/Scholastic, 2020. | Series: Xbooks
| Originally published: New York, NY : Scholastic, ©2012. | Audience: Ages 8-10. | Audience:
Grades 4-6. | Summary: "Book introduces the reader to flesh wounds"-- Provided by publisher.
Identifiers: LCCN 2020008046 | ISBN 9780531132319 (library binding) | ISBN 9780531132968 (paperback)
Subjects: LCSH: Staphylococcal infections--Juvenile literature. | Necrotizing fasciitis--Juvenile literature.
| Wounds and injuries--Infections--Juvenile literature.
Classification: LCC RC116.S8 P45 2020 | DDC 616.9/297--dc23
LC record available at https://lccn.loc.gov/2020008046

Printed in Johor Bahru, Malaysia   108

1 2 3 4 5 6 7 8 9 10 R 30 29 28 27 26 25 24 23 22 21

SCHOLASTIC, XBOOKS, and associated logos are trademarks and/or registered trademarks of Scholastic Inc.

Scholastic Inc., 557 Broadway, New York, NY 10012.

FLESH
WOUND

A Minor Injury
Takes a Deadly Turn

SHEA PHILLIPS

SCHOLASTIC

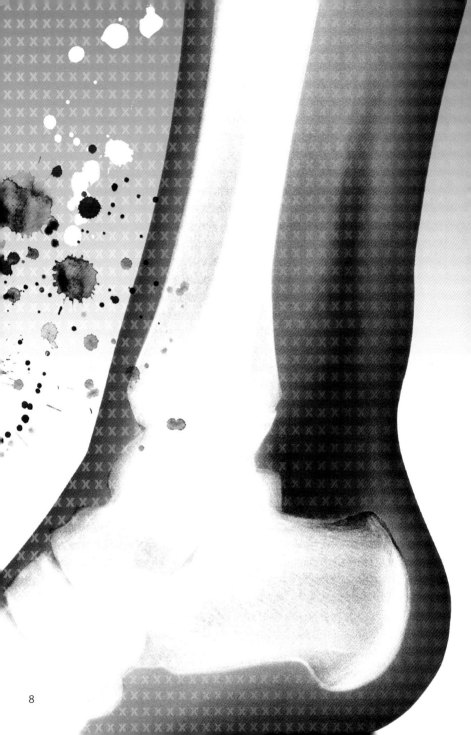

TABLE OF CONTENTS

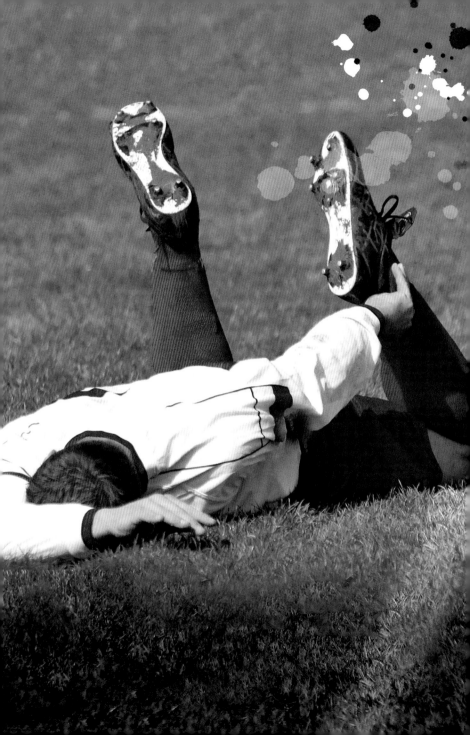

1

Foul!

For one soccer player, a little bruise is about to cause some big problems.

On Saturdays, Bo Salisbury played indoor soccer with teenagers from his church.

Salisbury was a 43-year-old postmaster in Nevada City, California. He usually played goalkeeper. In that position, he was used to getting bumped and bruised.

Salisbury was in the goal on May 9, 1998. It was a typical Saturday. He had a cold, but that wasn't going to slow him down. At one point during the game, players crowded around the goal, fighting for the ball.

Salisbury blocked a shot. But on his follow-through, the shooter accidentally kicked Salisbury on the left ankle. Salisbury limped off the field with a stinging bruise.

Just a Bruise?

The next day, the pain was worse. Salisbury took some aspirin. Then he had lunch at a local Chinese restaurant. By 2:00 P.M., his ankle was killing him. Salisbury went to the emergency room at a nearby hospital. A doctor examined Salisbury's ankle, which was turning red. The doctor decided it was just a nasty contusion, or bruise. He gave Salisbury some painkillers and sent him home.

By Monday morning, Salisbury was in terrible pain. He was sweating and felt sick to his stomach. His leg throbbed. He went to see his doctor, who sent him straight to the hospital. He told the doctors there that he felt like he was dying.

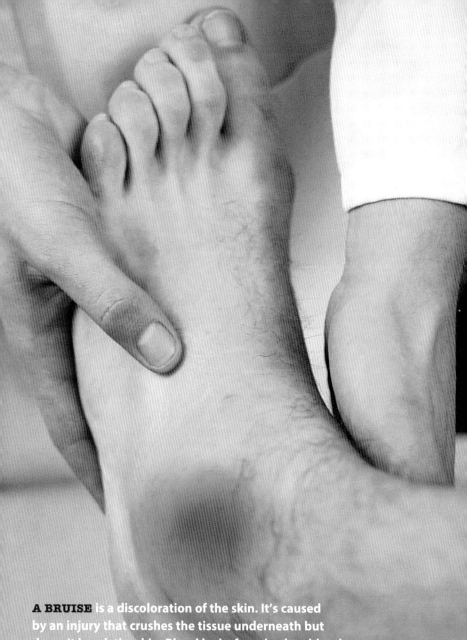

A BRUISE is a discoloration of the skin. It's caused by an injury that crushes the tissue underneath but doesn't break the skin. Blood leaks from broken blood vessels into the deep layer of skin, forming a bruise.

13

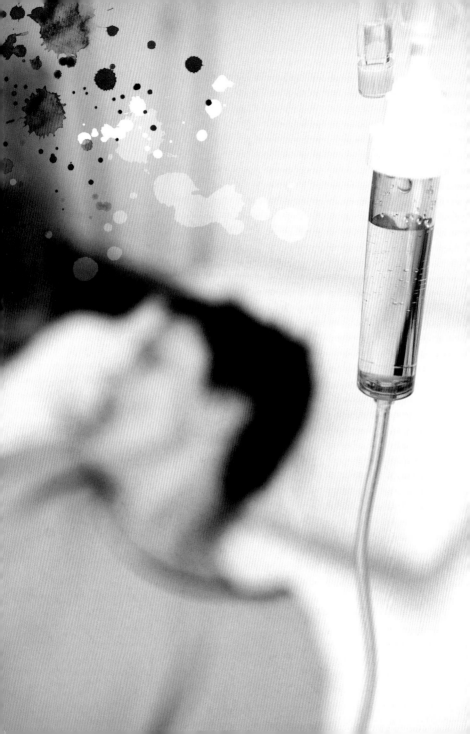

2

Critical Condition

Salisbury is failing fast. And his doctors are stumped.

Doctors at the hospital were concerned. It was clear that Bo Salisbury had more than a bruise. But what was causing his terrible symptoms? The doctors needed a diagnosis—and fast.

They took Salisbury's blood pressure. It was dropping quickly. They examined his leg. A blue-gray bruise had begun to spread out from his ankle. Doctors took a blood sample to test for a bacterial infection. While they waited for the results, they gave Salisbury an antibiotic drug to fight the infection.

Slipping Away

Salisbury continued to get worse. He slipped in and out of consciousness. He prepared himself to die. He told his teenage daughter not to cry and made her promise to study for her final exams. "There's nothing anyone can do for me now," he said.

Salisbury's doctors didn't know what to do. But they knew someone who might.

Salisbury would have to go to another hospital. The weather was too stormy for a helicopter, so Salisbury was wheeled to an ambulance. It raced to the University of California (UC) Davis Medical Center.

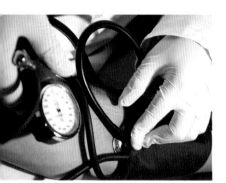

Meanwhile, like in a scene from a horror movie, the bruise continued to creep up Salisbury's leg.

FALLING BLOOD PRESSURE can be a sign that a patient is bleeding internally.

Constant Companions

Here are some frequently asked questions about bacteria.

What are bacteria? Bacteria are tiny, single-celled life-forms. They're the most common living things on Earth.

Where can you find bacteria? Everywhere! There are billions of bacteria all around you. They also live inside your body.

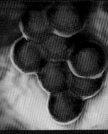

Staphylococcus aureus

Can bacteria hurt people? Most bacteria are harmless. But if conditions are just right (for them), some kinds of bacteria can cause big problems.

  Staphylococcus, or staph, lives on the skin and in the nose. When it gets under the outer layer of skin, it can cause a painful infection.

  Streptococcus, or strep, can cause throat infections. In rare cases it can get inside the skin. Then it causes a terrible disease called *necrotizing fasciitis* (NF), also known as flesh-eating disease.

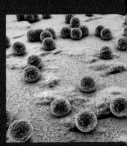

Streptococcus pyogenes

17

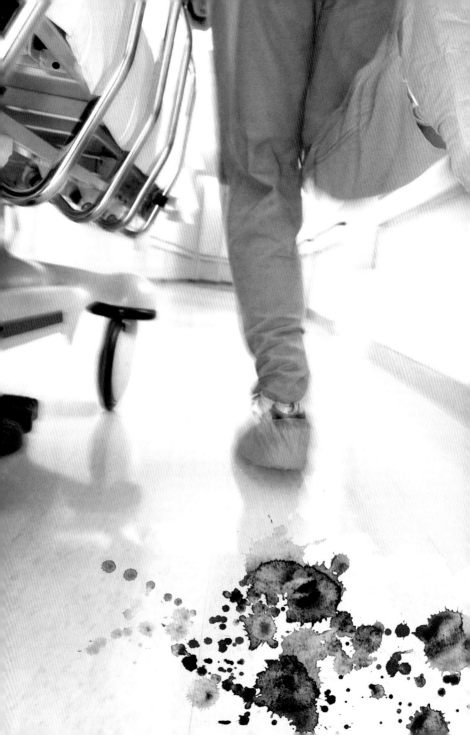

3

Life or Death

Dr. Susan Murin is Salisbury's last hope. Can she make a diagnosis before time runs out?

When he arrived at UC Davis Medical Center, Bo Salisbury was met by Dr. Susan Murin. She heads a team of doctors at the center's intensive care unit (ICU). That's the part of the hospital that treats the sickest patients. When they arrive, most of Murin's patients are close to death. But four out of five of them get better and walk out alive.

"Working in the ICU is never boring," says Dr.

Murin. "You see everything down here. You're more than a specialist. You have to be able to treat everything. You never know who is going to come through that door."

A Puzzling Case

Minutes after Salisbury arrived at the hospital, Murin and a team of doctors were at his bedside. One of the doctors was infectious-disease specialist Dr. Jeff Jones.

Salisbury was given oxygen and fluids. He could still talk, but he was failing fast.

Salisbury's case was confusing, even for Murin and Jones. Salisbury had kept in great shape. He had no history of illness. But in two days, he had gone from perfect health to the verge of death. What was wrong?

Murin carefully examined Salisbury's leg. The dark bruise was spreading slowly up his leg. To Murin, the leg looked like

DR. SUSAN MURIN is a specialist in critical care and internal medicine—the treatment of diseases of internal organs.

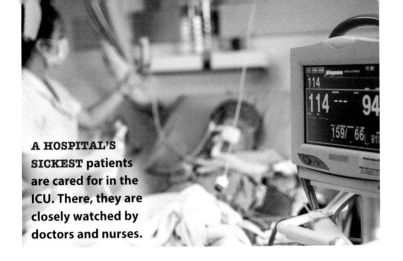

"rotten meat." The flesh felt cold to the touch. A normal infection would be red and warm. This leg wasn't getting blood. That led Murin to suspect that Salisbury had a blood clot. Perhaps the clot was keeping blood from flowing to his leg.

Murin ordered an ultrasound. This is a test that uses sound waves to create a picture of a person's insides. The image showed no blood clot. Then a call came from the hospital Salisbury had visited first. Salisbury's blood test results were in. They showed traces of a bacteria called *Streptococcus pyogenes*.

Murin had her diagnosis. Inside Salisbury's body, a strep infection was eating his flesh.

Lab Reports

Here's how lab technicians track down—and fight— an infection.

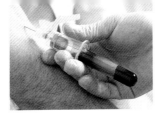

Drawing a
blood sample

Testing, Testing

Doctors take samples of a patient's body fluids—like blood, urine, and pus. Those samples are sent to a lab, where technicians test them.

Blood: Blood contains red blood cells and white blood cells. White blood cells help fight infections. So if a patient's white blood cell count is high, he might have an infection.

Urine: Dehydration occurs when there isn't enough fluid in the body. Infections can cause a person to become dehydrated. So urine is checked for signs of dehydration.

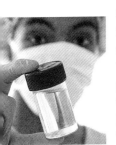

A urine
sample

Pus: The pus from a wound contains bacteria. Technicians take pus samples and try to make the bacteria grow. Then they perform chemical tests that identify the bacteria infecting the patient.

They also look at a sample under a microscope. *Streptococcus pyogenes* bacteria are sphere-shaped and grow in long chains. Staph bacteria look like clusters of grapes.

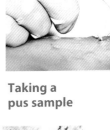

Taking a
pus sample

Treatment

Finally, the lab technicians look for an antibiotic that can kill the bacteria. They drip the antibiotics, one at a time, onto the bacteria. If the bacteria die, the technicians have found the right medicine.

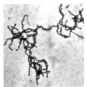

Streptococcus pyogenes

23

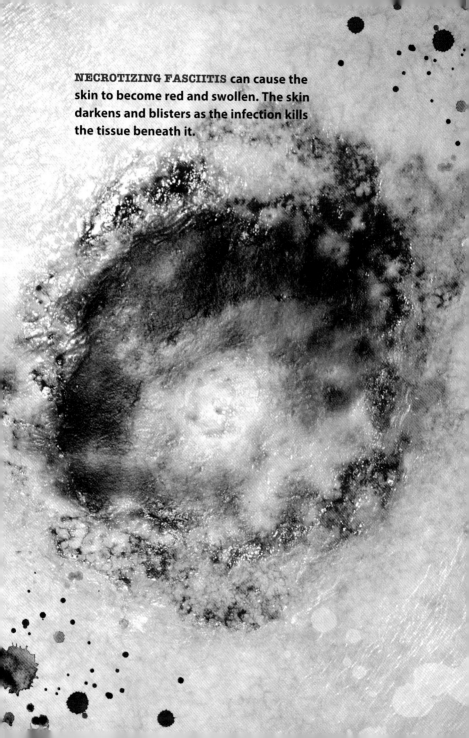

NECROTIZING FASCIITIS can cause the skin to become red and swollen. The skin darkens and blisters as the infection kills the tissue beneath it.

4

Brutal Bacteria

A deadly type of strep is eating Salisbury alive.

The test results proved to Dr. Murin and Dr. Jones that Salisbury had a life-threatening disease called necrotizing fasciitis (NF). NF is usually caused by the strep bacteria.

About 15 to 30 percent of all people carry strep in their bodies. In most people, strep is relatively harmless. It can cause common illnesses like strep throat or impetigo. Those diseases are easily cured with antibiotics. But in extremely rare cases, strep can lead to necrotizing fasciitis, a far more deadly disease. Only 500 to 1,500 Americans get NF every year. But more than one in five of them die from it.

Flesh Eater

People call NF the "flesh-eating disease" for good reason. Strep can consume human flesh.

Murin had seen NF only once before. But she knew how it killed. The strep bacteria produce toxins—poisons—in a patient's body. The toxins kill the soft tissue, or fascia, below the skin. The bacteria spread fast—about one inch (2.5 centimeters) an hour. And they kill tissue as they grow. If left untreated, NF can kill the patient.

Salisbury was already close to death. The antibiotics weren't working. His blood pressure kept dropping. He needed more and more oxygen. Murin was in a race against time.

"This thing travels fast," Salisbury said later. "In 72 hours, you kill it—or it kills you."

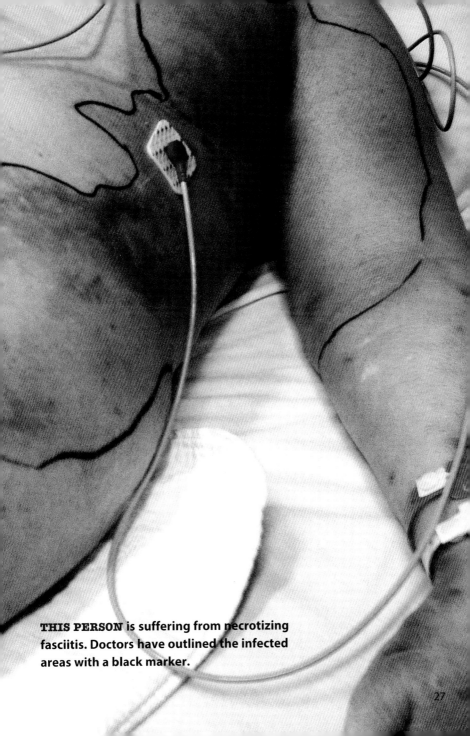

THIS PERSON is suffering from necrotizing fasciitis. Doctors have outlined the infected areas with a black marker.

From Mold to Medicine

Key Dates in the History of Infection

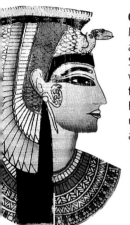

Good Molds
Many cultures use molds as medicine. For example, South American Indians wear moldy sandals to fight foot infections. The Egyptians and Chinese use molds to treat rashes and wounds.

Pasteur's Discovery
French scientist Louis Pasteur discovers that microorganisms cause wine and milk to spoil. This leads to the discovery that diseases can be caused by bacteria and other tiny germs. Those diseases can spread from person to person as germs are passed around.

3500–1500 BCE   **1300s**   **1870**

The Plague
The bubonic plague sweeps through Europe. The plague is a bacterial disease spread by fleas and rats. It can kill within a few days. More than 20 million people die.

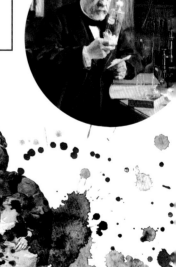

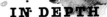

Cleaning Up
Doctors begin using sterilization to kill germs. They heat surgical instruments and wash their hands with soap. They wear masks and gowns to avoid spreading germs.

New Drugs
Researchers develop new antibiotics to fight staph. Methicillin, oxacillin, and vancomycin are the most effective. Vancomycin is usually given directly through the veins.

 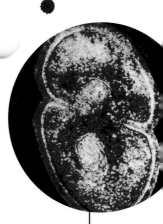

1890s	1928-29	1950s & 1960s	TODAY

Antibiotics Are Born
Scottish scientist Alexander Fleming discovers penicillin. It is the first modern antibiotic. During World War II (1939–1945), it is used to treat thousands of wounded soldiers.

New Superbugs
A new form of staph evolves that can't be killed by vancomycin. Experts say that new antibiotics are needed to stay one step ahead of deadly bacteria.

29

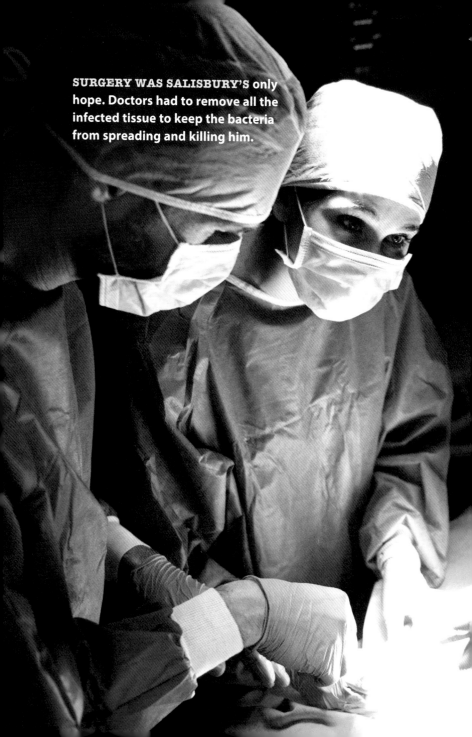

SURGERY WAS SALISBURY'S only hope. Doctors had to remove all the infected tissue to keep the bacteria from spreading and killing him.

5

Race Against Time

Surgeons race to strip away Salisbury's infected flesh.

Bo Salisbury had been in Dr. Murin's care for just two hours. She could see that he was getting sicker by the minute.

Salisbury was given antibiotics. But the drugs couldn't stop the infection that was racing through his body. Murin knew the infected flesh would have to be cut out of Salisbury's body. She called a surgeon and pleaded with him to operate on Salisbury.

The surgeon agreed. Still, Murin thought Salisbury's chances for recovery were poor. "I honestly thought he wasn't going to make it," she says. "He's such a nice guy. I was pulling for him. At the very least, I thought they'd have to amputate his leg."

Outracing Bacteria

Using special drugs, doctors put Salisbury into a coma. That's a state of deep unconsciousness. In a coma, his

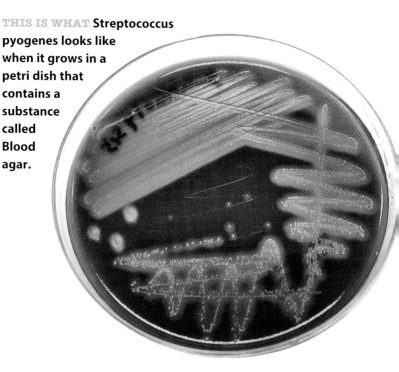

THIS IS WHAT Streptococcus pyogenes looks like when it grows in a petri dish that contains a substance called Blood agar.

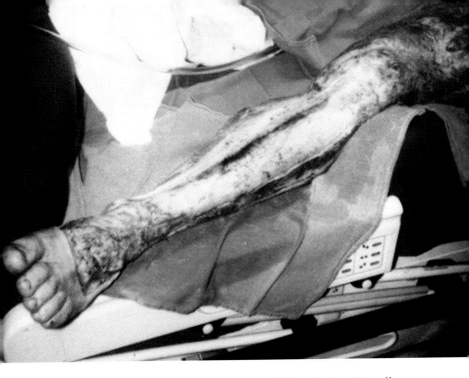

INFECTED TISSUE was removed from Salisbury's leg. "I'm all striped now," he said later.

body could handle the shock of what was coming next.

Surgeons raced against the bacteria as it spread up Salisbury's leg. The doctors cut into Salisbury's skin and began to slice off the infected tissue. In some places, they had to cut all the way down to the bone.

Finally, they were sure they had removed all of the bacteria. They also had to remove most of the flesh from Salisbury's toes to his hip. But when Salisbury left the operating room, he still had his leg—and his life.

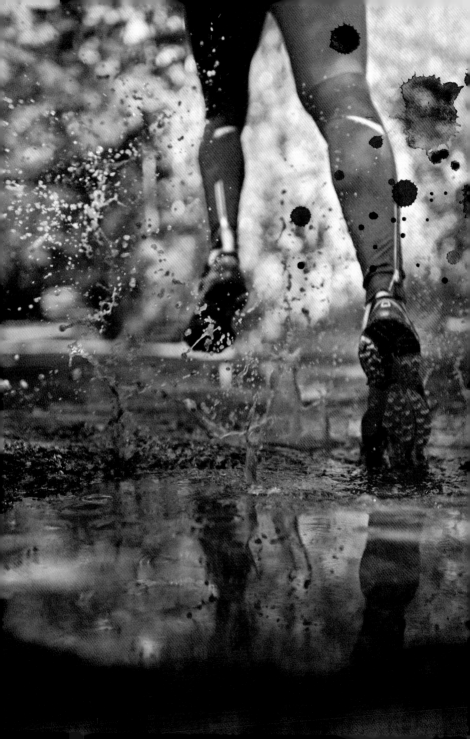

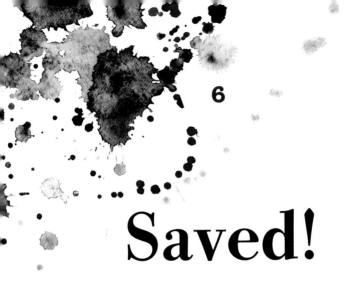

6

Saved!

**Surviving the killer bacteria
is just the first step on Salisbury's
long road to recovery.**

Bo Salisbury woke up from the coma 10 days later. Doctors had spent a week replacing the flesh on his leg with skin grafts. They'd peeled flesh from other parts of Salisbury's body. Then they sewed the flesh onto his leg. Salisbury felt like he had been skinned alive. "I'm all striped now," he jokes. "People stare at me when I wear shorts."

In all, Salisbury underwent eight skin grafts. The treatments left him weak and depressed.

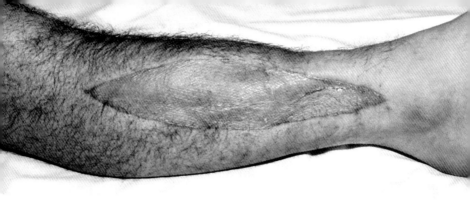

A SKIN GRAFT on a patient's leg. Skin grafts are used to replace skin that has been destroyed by infections, burns, or other injuries.

But little by little, Salisbury recovered. He started rehabilitation to strengthen his body. He had to re-learn how to do everyday activities. After five months, Salisbury was finally able to go home from the hospital.

Eventually, Salisbury was able to run a few miles a day. He even competed in a five-kilometer (3-mile) race. Some Saturdays, you can still find him playing goalie for his church soccer team.

Medical Mysteries

Bo Salisbury sometimes wonders how he got such a rare disease. Strep has no effect on some people, but it can be deadly for others. Even Dr. Murin can't explain exactly why. "There are so many mysteries in medicine that we still don't understand," she says. **X**

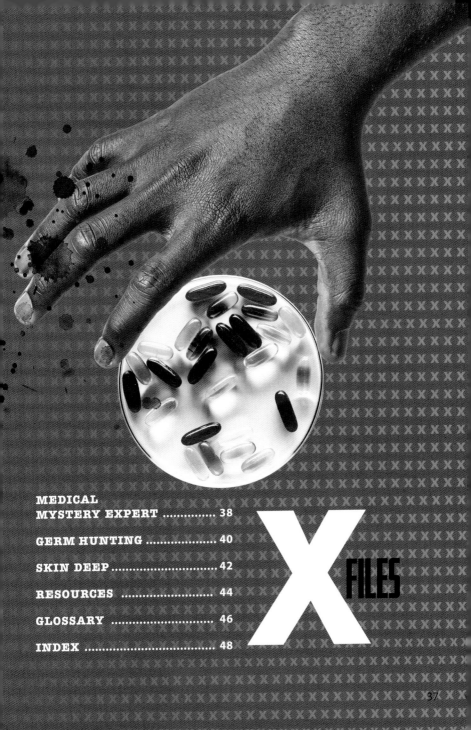

X FILES

Medical Mystery Expert

Dr. Rekha Murthy is a disease detective.

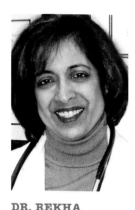

DR. REKHA MURTHY has been a professor of clinical medicine at the University of California at Los Angeles. She has also worked as an infectious disease specialist at Cedars-Sinai Hospital in L.A.

How did you become an infectious disease specialist?

MURTHY: After I graduated from college, I went to medical school. Then I worked three years as a resident in internal medicine.

What got you interested in infectious diseases?

MURTHY: I got very interested in fields like cancer and infectious disease because you have to know a lot about all the body systems. I also loved the detective work that infectious disease often requires.

Describe a typical day at your job.

MURTHY: I begin by seeing patients. Other doctors ask for my advice on cases concerning infection and fever. I help identify the disease. I guide the medical team about what tests to order. I also advise on which treatments and antibiotics to administer. I give on-the-job training to doctors, medical students, nurses, and staff. I also do research and work with trainees.

What happens after work?

MURTHY: I bring medical journals home and look up information online. I network with colleagues to discuss complicated cases. Medicine moves so fast, especially in my field. We have to get the information as quickly as possible and be a resource to the other staff in the hospital.

What do you like most about your work?

MURTHY: I like that it's never the same. I always feel like I'm learning. And I really feel like I am making a difference by sharing information and participating with patient care.

What advice do you have for young people who are interested in this field?

MURTHY: Develop good interpersonal skills. You need to communicate with patients in a compassionate manner. You also need to be able to be seen as a leader.

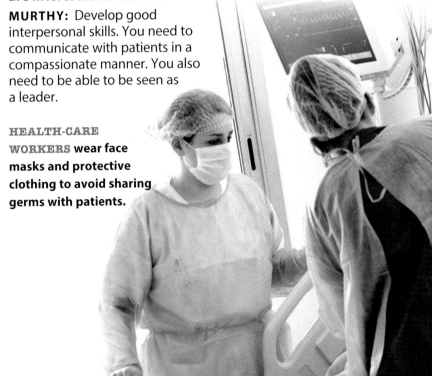

HEALTH-CARE WORKERS **wear face masks and protective clothing to avoid sharing germs with patients.**

Germ Hunting

Check out an infectious disease specialist's tools of the trade.

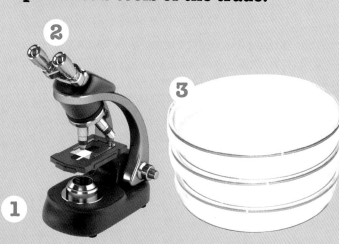

1 Syringe and needle Nurses and doctors use a syringe and needle to inject medicine into patients. These are also used to withdraw blood and other fluids from the body.

2 Microscope Lab technicians use microscopes to look for bacteria in fluid samples taken from patients.

3 Petri dishes Lab techs store bacteria samples in these dishes. They keep them at body temperature—about 98.6 degrees Fahrenheit (37 degrees Celsius)—so the bacteria will grow.

4 Slide Lab techs smear this thin piece of glass with a fluid sample. The slide fits under the microscope lens.

5 X-ray machine This device uses high-energy beams to create images of the inside of a body. The X-rays can show damage that an infection has done to tissues and bones.

Skin Deep

Here's a close-up look at some nasty skin infections.

CELLULITIS

NECROTIZING FASCIITIS

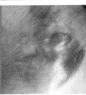

IMPETIGO

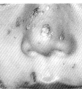

BOILS

FOLLICULITIS

SCALDED SKIN SYNDROME

SCARLET FEVER

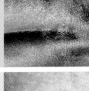

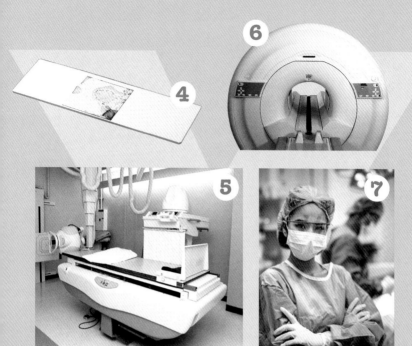

6 MRI This device uses radio waves to take highly detailed pictures of a patient's insides. "MRI" stands for *magnetic resonance imaging*.

7 Universal precautions

Handling body fluids from infected people is dangerous. So health-care workers follow a set of rules called universal precautions.

They include:

- using only sterilized, disposable needles and syringes
- immediately throwing away needles in a safe container
- washing hands with soap and water before and after working with patients
- using protection such as gloves, gowns, aprons, masks, and goggles
- sterilizing instruments and other equipment

INDEX

postmaster (POHST-mass-tur) *noun* the head of a post office

pus (PUHSS) *noun* a thick, yellow liquid produced in infected tissue; it is made of dead white blood cells, bacteria, and tissue cells

necrotizing fasciitis (NEK-roh-tye-zing fah-shee-EYE-tiss) *noun* an infection that destroys skin and the tissue underneath; it is usually caused by *Streptococcus pyogenes*

rehabilitation (ree-huh-bil-ih-TAY-shun) *noun* the process of recovering from an illness or injury

skin graft (SKIN GRAFT) *noun* transplanted skin from one part of the body to replace skin in a damaged area

staph (STAF) *noun* a common bacteria carried on skin and in noses; it's short for *Staphylococcus*

sterilization (ster-uhl-ih-ZAY-shun) *noun* the process of cleaning something to make it free of bacteria and other microorganisms

strep (STREP) *noun* a common bacteria that can cause skin infections, strep throat, and scarlet fever; it's short for *Streptococcus*

Streptococcus pyogenes (strep-tuh-COK-us PYE-oh-jeenz) *noun* the type of strep that most often causes necro-tizing fasciitis

symptom (SIMP-tuhm) *noun* a sign of an illness

throbbing (THROB-ing) *adjective* describing pain that comes in a series of regular beats

tissue (TISH-oo) *noun* in an animal or plant, a group of cells that perform the same task; the four basic types of tissue in an animal are connective tissue, muscle tissue, nervous tissue, and epithelial tissue

ultrasound (UHL-truh-sound) *noun* a test that uses sound waves to create an image of the inside of the body

toxin (TOK-sin) *noun* a poisonous substance produced by a microorganism that causes disease when absorbed by body tissue

GLOSSARY

amputate (AM-pyuh-tate) *verb* to cut off a body part, usually because it is damaged or diseased

antibiotic (an-tee-bye-OT-ik) *noun* a drug that kills harmful bacteria

bacteria (bak-TEER-ee-ah) *noun* single-celled life-forms, some of which can cause disease in humans or other animals

blood clot (BLUHD CLOT) *noun* a mass of thickened blood

blood pressure (BLUHD PRESH-ur) *noun* a measure of how hard blood is pushing against blood vessel walls

coma (KOH-muh) *noun* a state of deep unconsciousness, usually caused by a disease or injury

connective tissues (kuh-NEK-tiv TISH-ooz) *noun* groups of cells, such as bone marrow, tendons, and cartilage, that provide structure and support within an animal body

consciousness (KON-shuhss-ness) *noun* the state of being awake and able to think and perceive

contusion (kon-TOO-shun) *noun* an injury that doesn't break the skin but causes discoloration; a bruise

dehydration (dee-hye-DRAY-shun) *noun* a dangerous lack of water in the body

diagnosis (di-ag-NOH-sis) *noun* the identification of a condition or disease

fascia (FA-shee-uh) *noun* a sheet of connective tissue separating or keeping together organs and muscles

impetigo (im-peh-TYE-go) *noun* a staph or strep infection that causes pimple-like sores

infectious disease specialist (in-FEK-shuhss duh-ZEEZ SPESH-uh-list) *noun* a doctor who specializes in diagnosing and treating all kinds of infections

intravenous (in-tra-VEE-nis) *adjective* entering directly into a vein

microorganism (mye-kroh-OR-guh-niz-uhm) *noun* a living thing that is too small to be seen without a microscope

painkiller (PAYN-kil-ur) *noun* medicine taken to stop pain

FICTION

Cooney, Caroline B. *Code Orange.*
New York: Delacorte Press, 2005.

Dahme, Joanne. *The Plague.*
Philadelphia: Running Press, 2009.

Hayles, Marsha. *Breathing Room.*
New York: Square Fish, 2013.

Holm, Jennifer. *Squish #7: Deadly
Disease of Doom.* New York: Random
House, 2015.

Koch, Falynn. *Plagues: The
Microscopic Battlefield (Science
Comics).* New York: First Second,
2017.

Pearson, Mary E. *The Adoration
of Jenna Fox.* New York: Henry
Holt, 2008.

Here's a selection of books for more information about bacteria and infectious diseases.

NONFICTION

Biskup, Agnieszka Jòzefina. *The Surprising World of Bacteria with Max Axiom, Super Scientist: 4D an Augmented Reading Science Experience (Graphic Science 4D).* North Mankato, Minnesota: Capstone, 2016.

DiConsiglio, John. *Superbugs (Hot Topics).* Portsmouth, New Hampshire: Heinemann, 2012.

Eamer, Claire. *Inside Your Insides: A Guide to the Microbes That Call You Home.* Toronto: Kids Can Press, 2016.

Gardy, Jennifer. *It's Catching: The Infectious World of Germs and Microbes.* Toronto: Owlkids, 2014.

Mould, Steve. *The Bacteria Book: The Big World of Really Tiny Microbes.* London: DK Children, 2018.

Orr, Tamra. *Antibiotics (A True Book).* New York: Scholastic, 2016.

Rooney, Anne. *You Wouldn't Want to Live Without Antibiotics!* New York: Scholastic, 2014.

Tilden, Thomasine E. *Help! What's Eating My Flesh: Runaway Staph and Strep Infections! (24/7: Science Behind the Scenes: Medical Files).* New York: Scholastic, 2007.

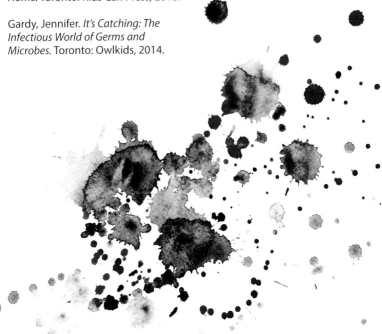

Cause and Symptoms	Treatment
Caused by staph or strep. It is a swelling of the skin and the connective tissues underneath. Cellulitis usually forms on the upper body, arms, or legs. Skin turns painful, red, and tender. Swelling can blister and turn into a scab.	Oral or intravenous (IV) antibiotics
NF is usually caused by a rare kind of strep bacteria. It's an infection that destroys skin and soft tissue. NF can be fatal.	Immediate hospitalization; antibiotics to kill the bacteria; surgery to cut out infected and dead tissue
A staph or strep infection. It causes pimple-like sores, often around the nose and mouth. The blisters can burst, ooze, and then form a thick crust. The infection can itch and spread.	Ointment; antibiotics in some cases
Usually caused by staph. Swollen red sores fill with pus. The sores may appear anywhere on the body.	Applying a warm, wet cloth. In some cases, boils may need to be operated on and drained of pus.
Tiny whitehead pimples often caused by staph. They form at the base of hair shafts. They are often found on women who wear their hair tightly pulled back.	Usually clears on its own in one week
Staph infection that turns into a rash that blisters and then causes the skin to peel off. It commonly affects children under age five.	Antibiotics; ointment
Rash made up of tiny red pinpoints. It can follow a case of strep throat. It begins as a red rash on the neck and chest. It may spread around the body.	Antibiotics